Ehlers Danlos Syndrome
With Liberty the Dog,
an Emotional Support Dog,
Helps You Explain
Ehlers Danlos Syndrome
to Others.

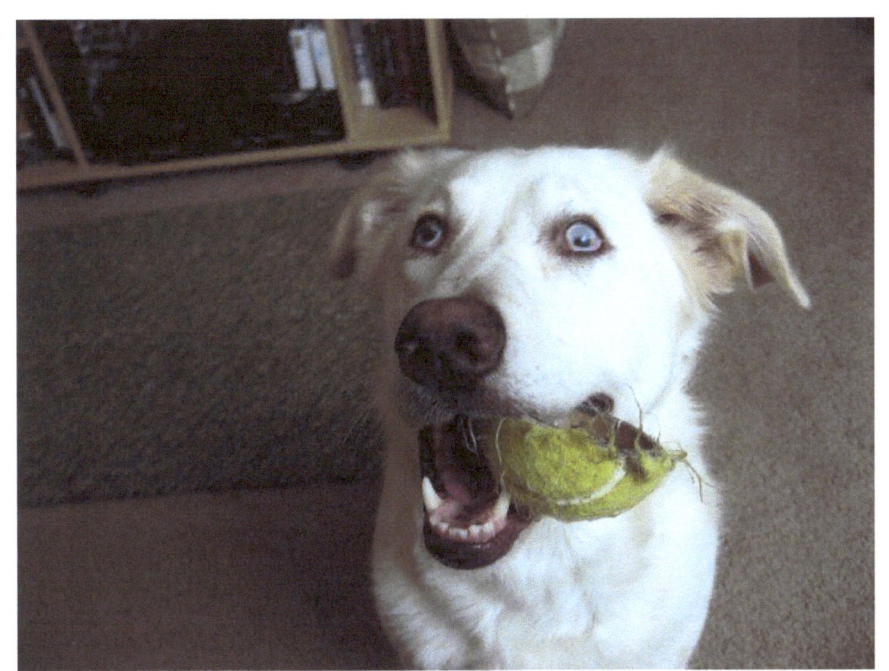

Ehlers Danlos Syndrome
With Liberty the Dog,
an Emotional Support Dog,
Helps You Explain
Ehlers Danlos Syndrome
to Others.

Written by and Photographs by
Amy Dee Hosp
Copyright © 2018

The Liberty of It All
With Genes That Don't Fit ©

Pete & Gracie Publishing

Title ID: 1723438138
ISBN-13: 9781723438134

Isaiah 41:10

So do not fear, for I am with you;
do not be dismayed, for I am your God.
I will strengthen you and help you;
I will uphold you with my righteous right hand.

New International Version

My name is
Liberty Ufan Mi [OU Fahn ME].
Ufan Mi means "My Friend"
in the African Ibibio language.
I was born on January 15, 2007.

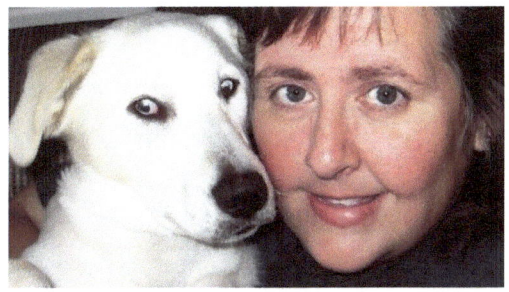

My human Mommy is my best friend and
I love her very much.
She loves me very much also.
I do silly things all the
time that my Mommy laughs at.

I am part Labrador retriever
and part heeler. I have blue eyes
with pupils that are
shaped kind of funny.
The pupils in my eyes are in the
bottom of my eyes instead
of in the center of my eyes.
Also, my pupils are not round like
other dogs, they are shaped funny.
In my right eye there is a green spot.
My eyes look like this because I am what is called
a Double Merle dog.
I am white with blonde patches
here and there.

My eyes look different
than other dog's eyes

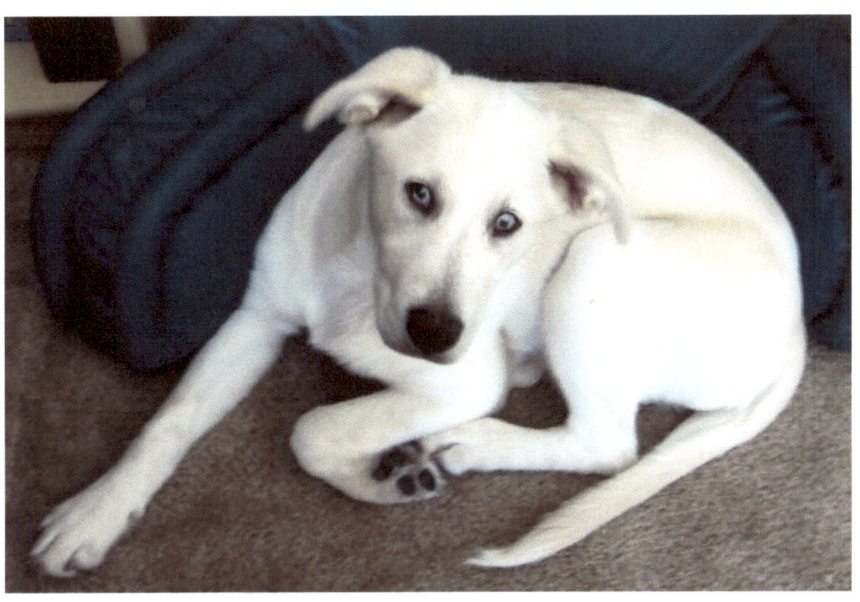

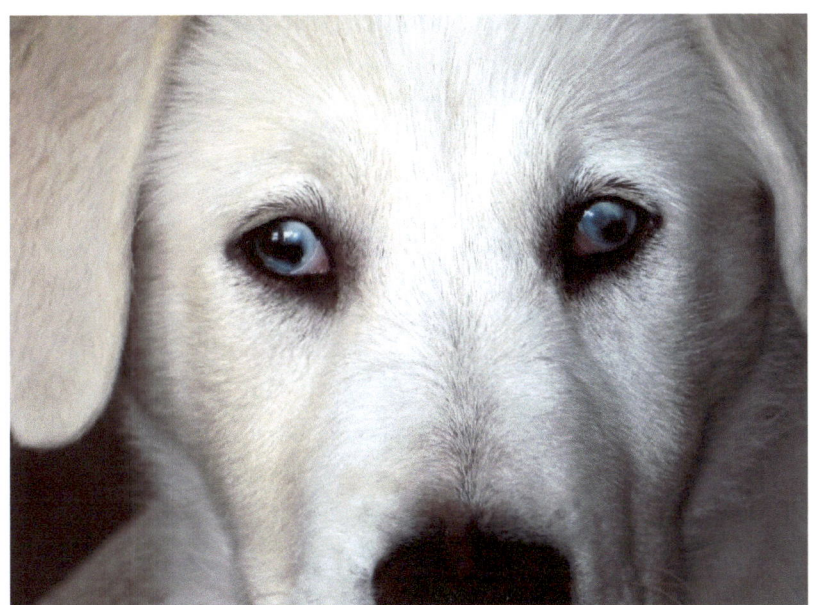

but it is not the only thing
that is different about me.

I
    have
        a
            genetic
                disorder
                    called
                        Ehlers Danlos Syndrome.

This is a disorder that can be common in dogs but in people it is more uncommon to have it.

Can you believe that people and horses and dogs could have Ehlers Danlos Syndrome?

Ehlers Danlos Syndrome, EDS for short, is something that you are born with because one of your parents, or sometimes both of your parents also have it.

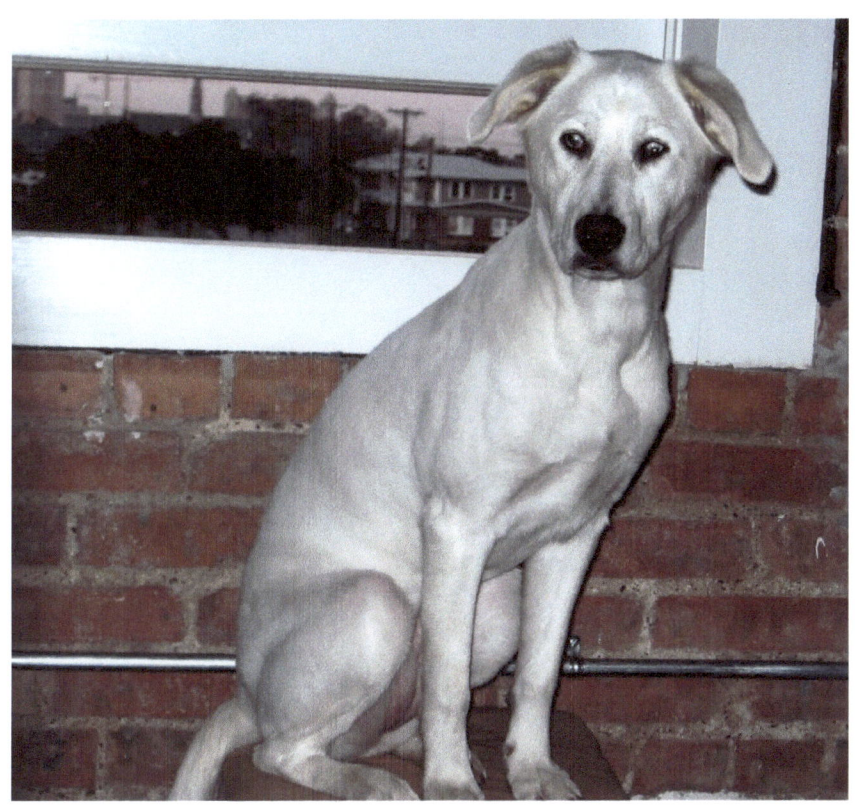

To have Ehlers Danlos means that you make collagen that doesn't work as well as other people and dog's collagen.

Your body is made up of almost all collagen.

Eighty percent of
your body is made from collagen
which is like glue that holds
your body together.

Making good collagen is very important.
Without good collagen our bodies fall apart.
A body without good collagen is like a house you build out of sticks with glue that doesn't do its job. A stick house held together with bad glue will not stay together,
it will just fall apart.

One of the jobs of the glue in our bodies is to hold joints together. If the glue, that is collagen, doesn't work, then the muscles and tendons and ligaments are not strong enough to hold the joints together.

When the collagen in our bodies doesn't work well our joints get overstretched which causes the joints to move, or pop, out of place. Sometimes a joint that has come out of place can be described as the bone coming out of joint.
When this happens, it is called a dislocated joint.

Because people with EDS don't make good collagen they can bend parts of their body more than other people. That means that if you have EDS you can bend your fingers and toes and wrists and neck and back and elbows and knees and hips beyond what people without EDS can do.

If you can bend your joints more than most people be very careful not to do it on purpose. Sometimes it is fun to show how much we can bend our joints. If we show off how much we can bend our joints it can cause harm and pain to your joints. Some people call this being doubled jointed but there is really no such thing as being doubled jointed.

I can bend my joints more than other dogs without EDS because my collagen doesn't work very well. I'm not doing this on purpose, this is just how my joints are naturally.

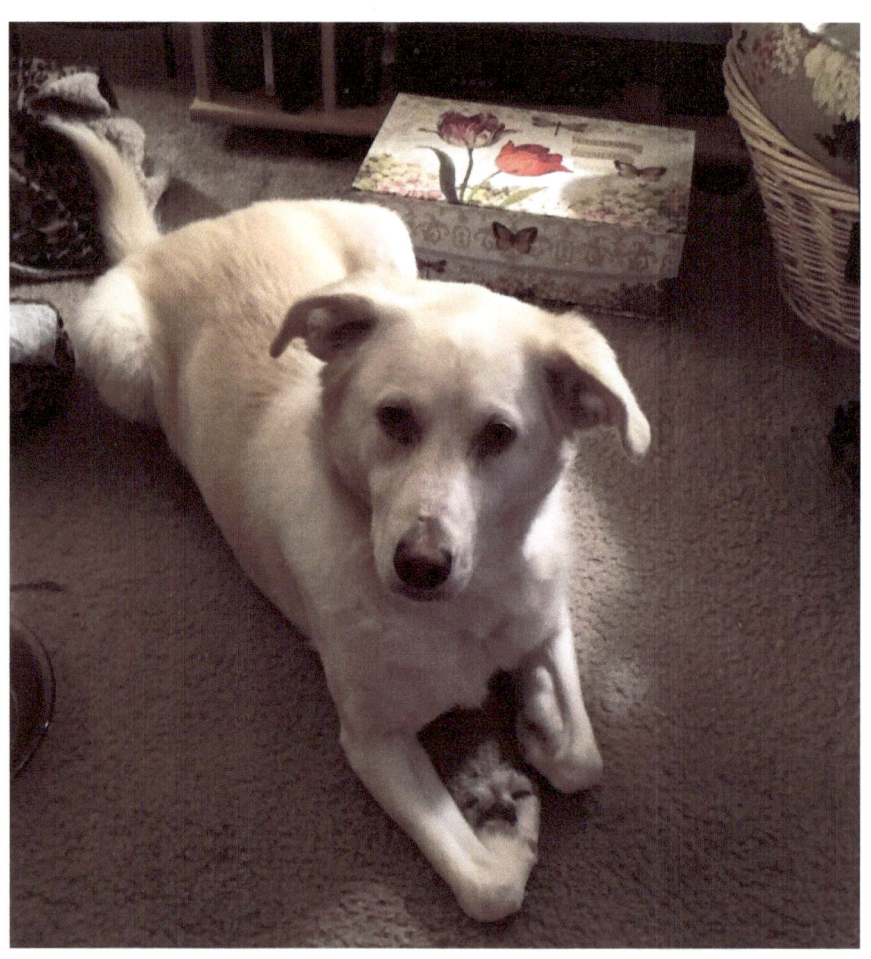

Can you see how bendy my joints are?

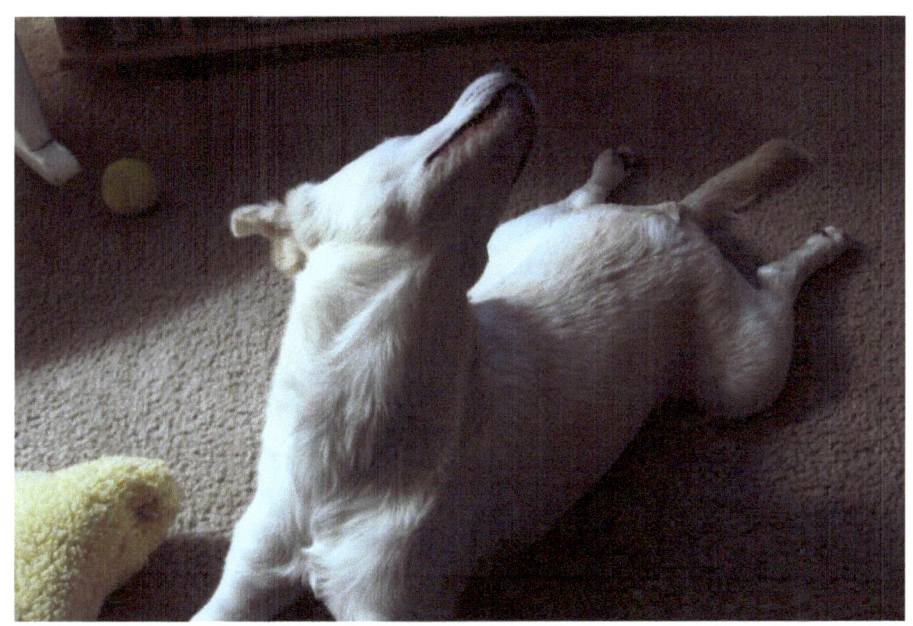

My neck is bendy too!

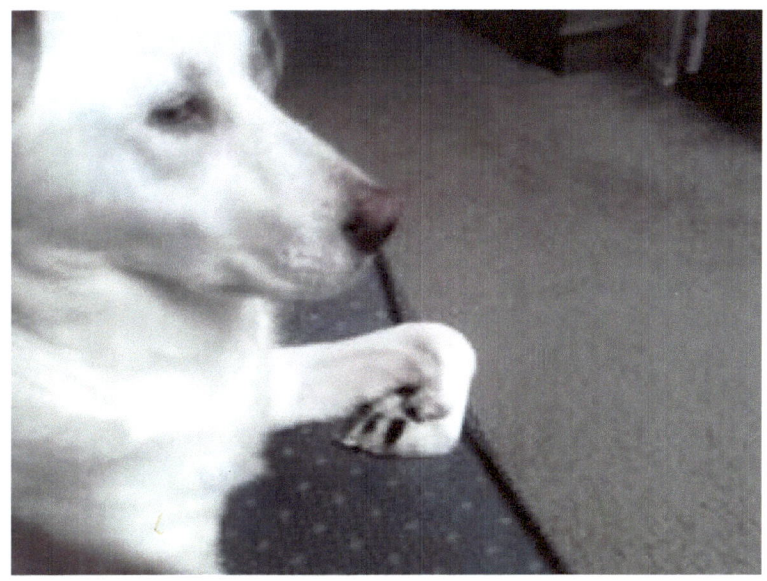

This is
     also
          called
               being
                    flexible.

Researchers and doctors are working on finding a way to help the body make better collagen but so far no one has found anything that helps.

It's important to find help because having EDS causes your body to have a lot a pain and it causes you to have a hard time doing things like running and playing and cleaning your room and doing housework.

EDS can even cause homework to be hard to do. Often, people with EDS have a hard time holding their pencil correctly, and sometimes people with EDS have so much pain that it is hard to concentrate on schoolwork.

Sometimes people who have EDS feel left out of activities because the activities may cause harm to their joints. This can cause people to feel lonely.

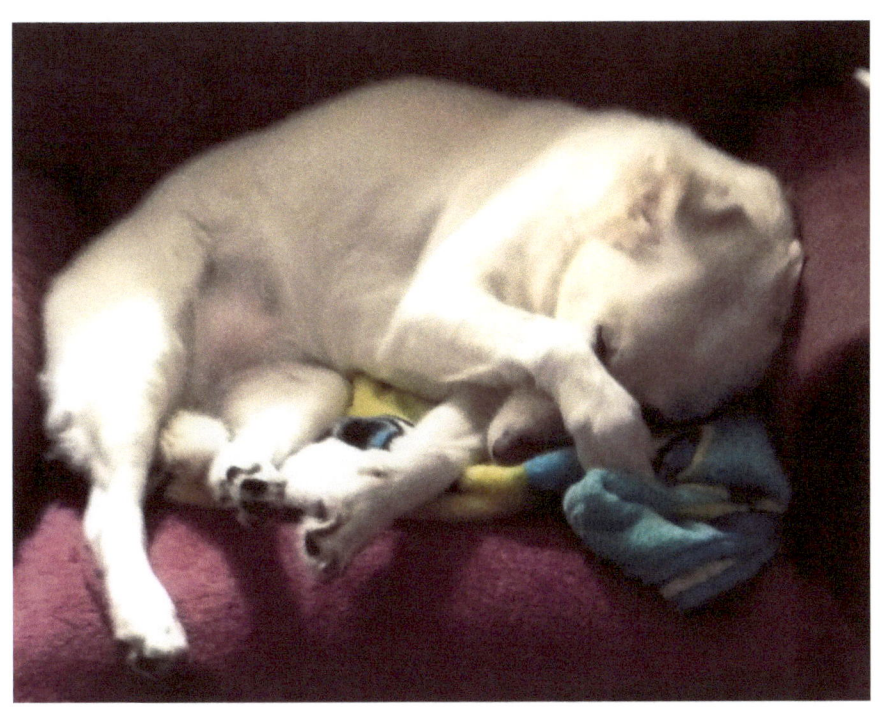

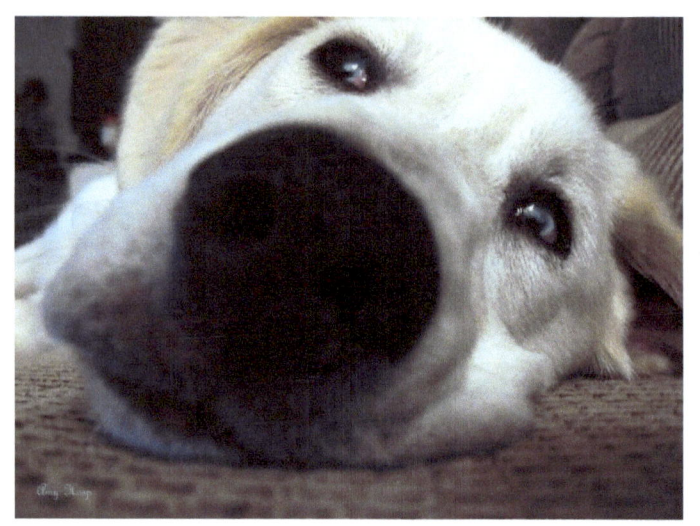

If you make a mess while playing with your toys it can be hard to clean. With EDS bending over and picking things up can sometimes cause you to be dizzy and cause pain in your joints.

People with EDS need to be very careful to not hold too many things at one time so that they will not hurt the joints in their shoulders, elbows, wrists, hips and back.

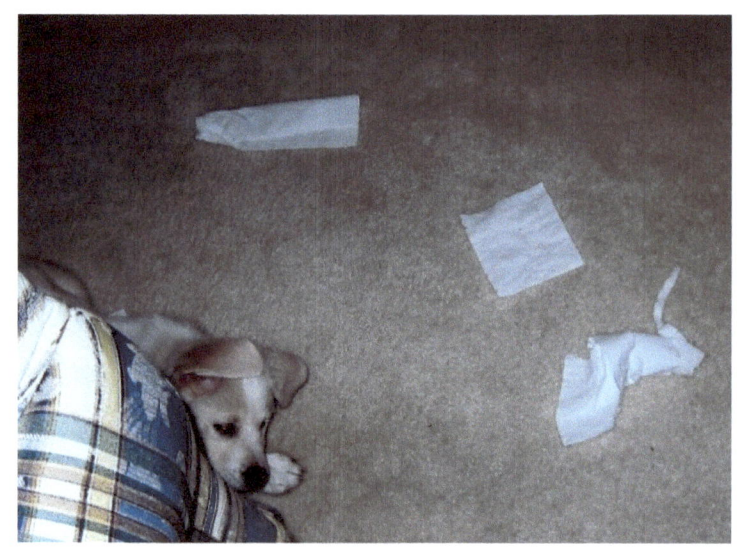

The pain happens because of the way the joints and muscles and ligaments and tendons get overstretched when you move around and pick up heavy things.

I have to tell you that there is something very special about me having EDS.

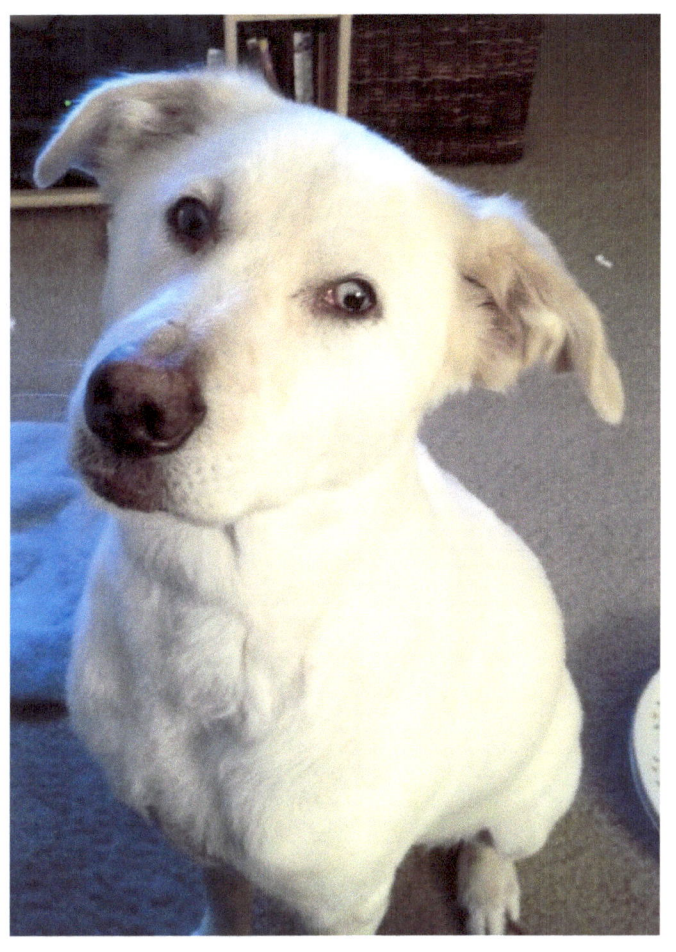

My Mommy has EDS also.

That is special because she and I have the same genetic disorder so it is really easy for us to understand each other about why we don't feel good on some days.

When my Mommy was a puppy,

oops, I mean a little girl,

she was bendy like me.

She's still bendy as an adult.

That's my Mommy when she was a kid.

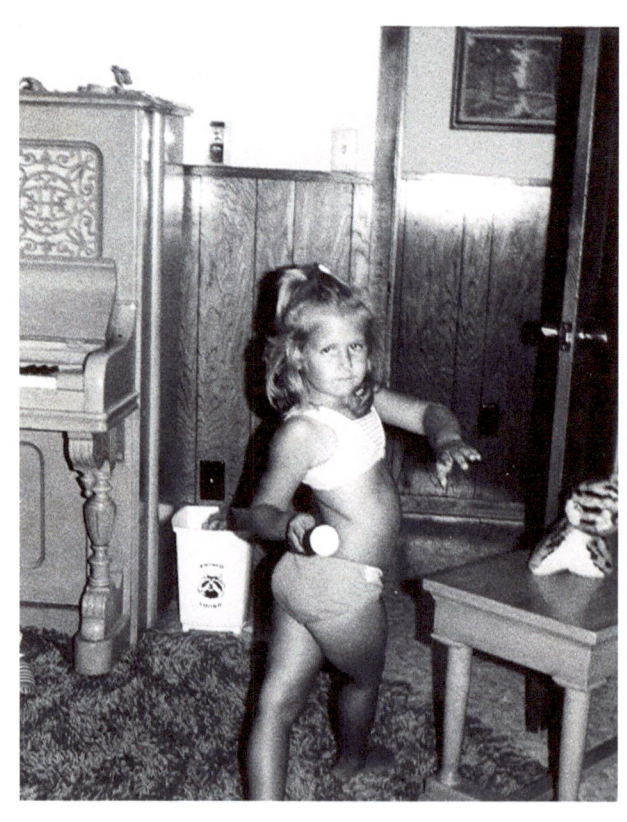

There are
several different types of
Ehlers Danlos Syndrome.

The type that my Mommy has is called
Classical Type I
sometimes called just
Classical Type.

I don't know the name of the type
that I have but my symptoms
and my Mommy's symptoms
are very much alike.

We both have very soft skin
that feels like baby's skin.
It feels velvety and it looks like a
young persons or a puppy's skin.
Even though I am older now,
my skin on my tummy is still just as
soft as when I was a puppy.

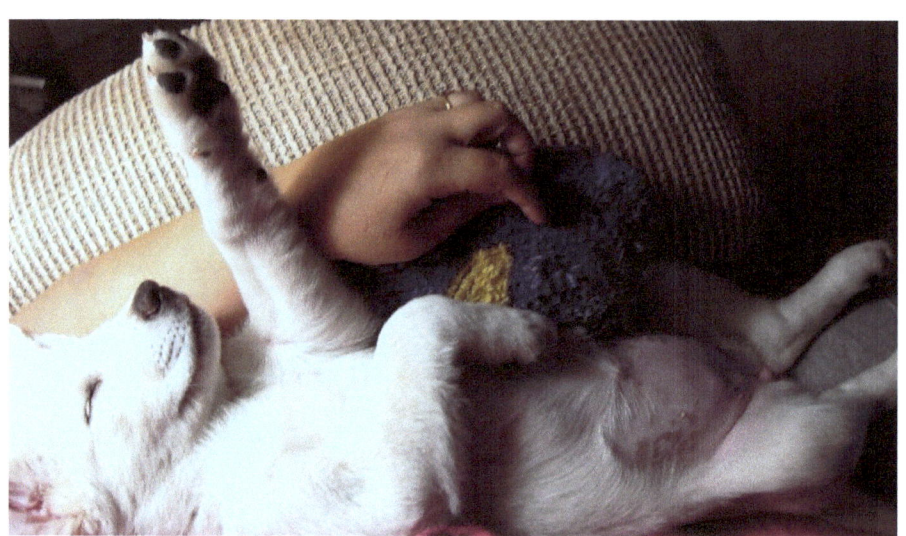

With such soft skin we have to be
careful because our skin pulls apart easily.
It is very easy to cut our skin when we
are playing. We have to be extra careful
to watch out for sharp things.
We also get bruises very easily.

Sometimes when I jump on Mommy or step on her she gets bruises and they turn purple and green. I don't mean to give Mommy bruises but it is just part of what is wrong with her body. She never gets mad at me when that happens.

Another symptom that we have that is the same is bendy joints. People and dogs without EDS have ligaments and tendons that are like a rubber band. When you pull a rubber band and let go of it, it snaps right back to the way it always is.

Ligaments and tendons are what hold our joints and bones together.

People and dogs
that have EDS have ligaments
and tendons and muscles that
are like chewing gum.
When you chew
your gum and then
take it out of your
mouth and pull on the gum
and let it go, after doing that
a lot of times, it does not
go back to the way it was
before you pulled on it, it stays
stretched out and if you pull on it too
many times, it just pulls right apart.

Because my joints and my Mommy's joints are like chewing gum,
if they get pulled on too many times, one day they will not be
able to stay in place and we may have to have an
operation to fix them.

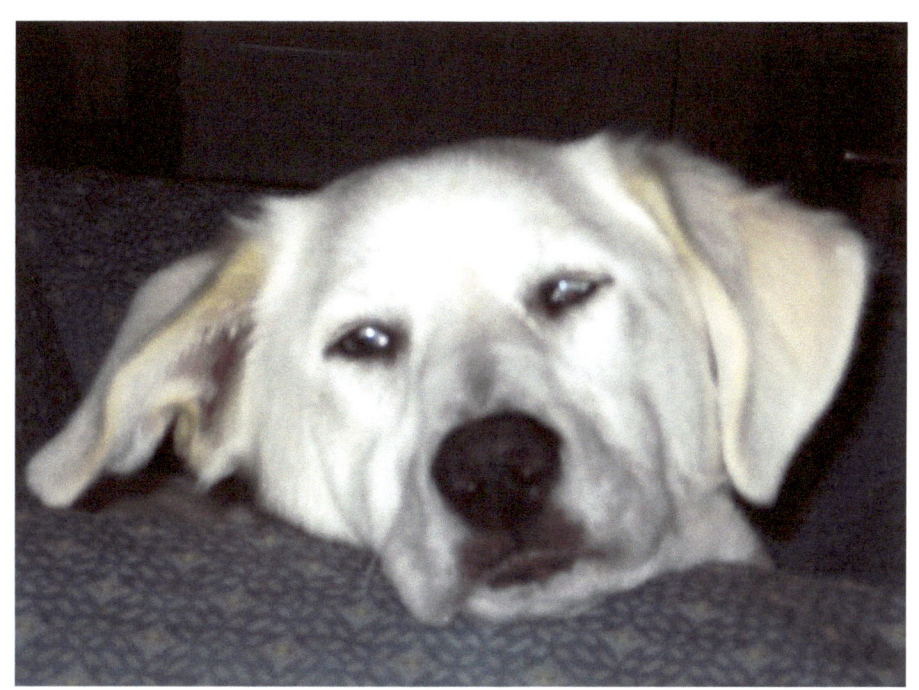

Sometimes people with EDS need to use crutches or a cane or a walker or a wheelchair to get around.

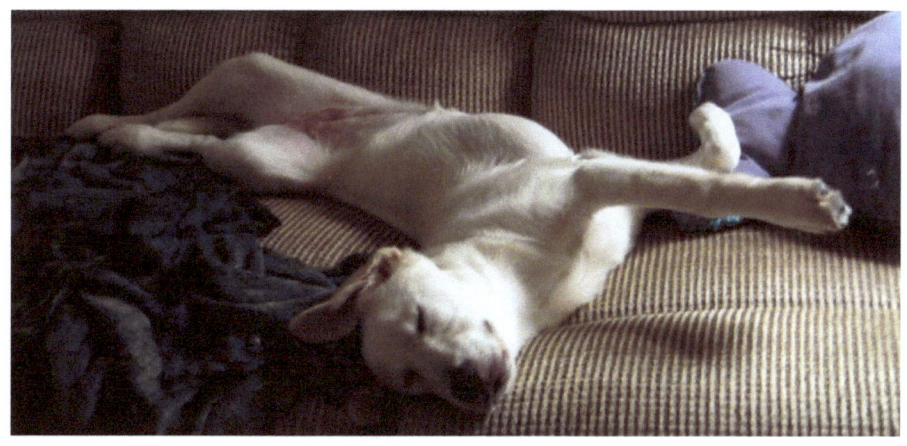

Being stretchy helps you really spread out for a nap!

Having bendy joints means
that it is very easy to hurt our joints.
We need to be careful when we are
playing not to pull or jump
too much so that we don't
injure our joints.

This play is too rough. I may dislocate a
joint or cut my skin.

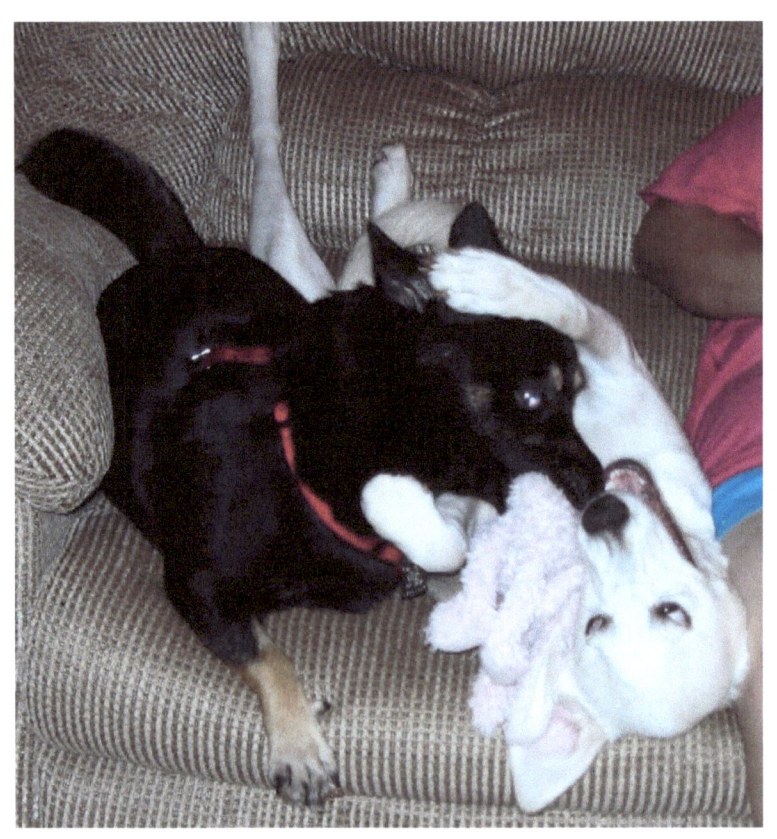

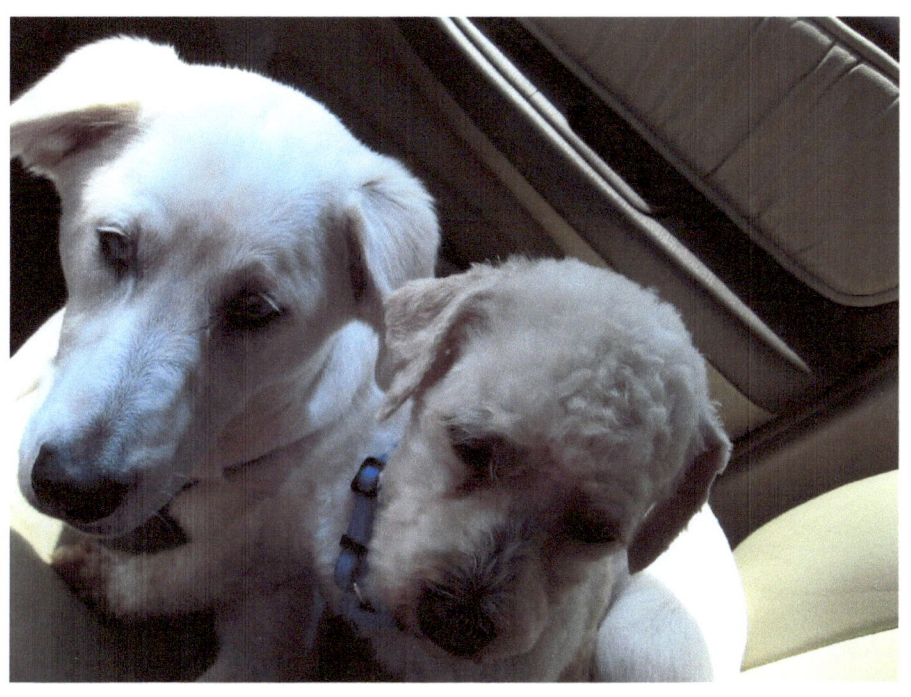

Sometimes it's just better to watch a movie,
read a book, or play a game
where we can sit still while we play.

My joints pop and sometimes get dislocated when
I am playing. A joint that pops is not
the same as a joint getting dislocated.
Mommy's joints get dislocated sometimes
when we are playing and it hurts super
bad so we have to stop playing and
rest for a while instead.

Once in a while I
have to go to the emergency
room with Mommy because
she gets hurt enough to have a
doctor check out her joints.
She doesn't play as much as she used to.
Her injuries come mostly from just doing everyday things.

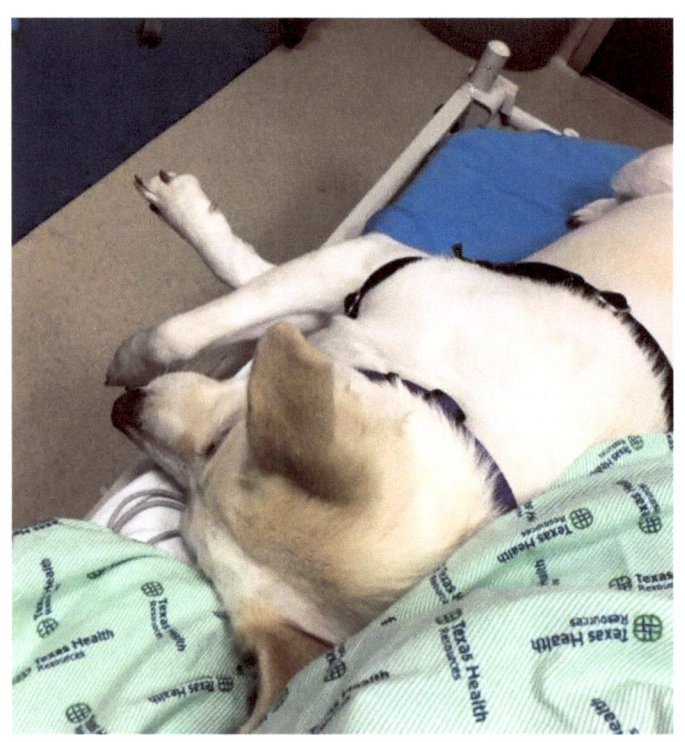

I
   love
        to
            run
                and
                    play

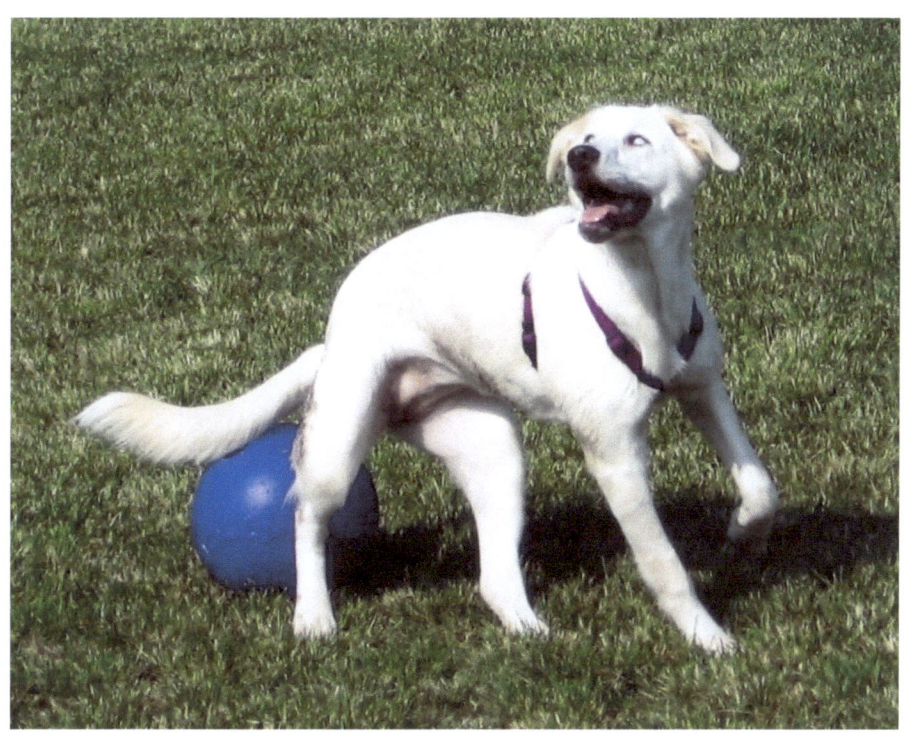

But ....

I get tired after just a few minutes of playing. My body is having to work hard to keep my joints from getting hurt.

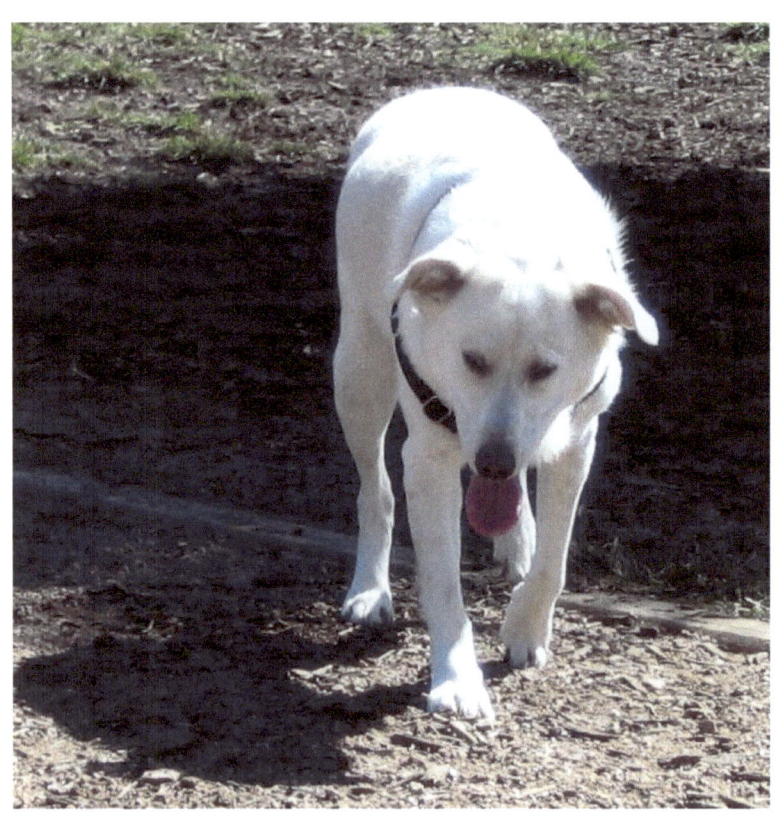

It is important to know how to protect your joints when you are playing with your friends and family and when you are playing sports.

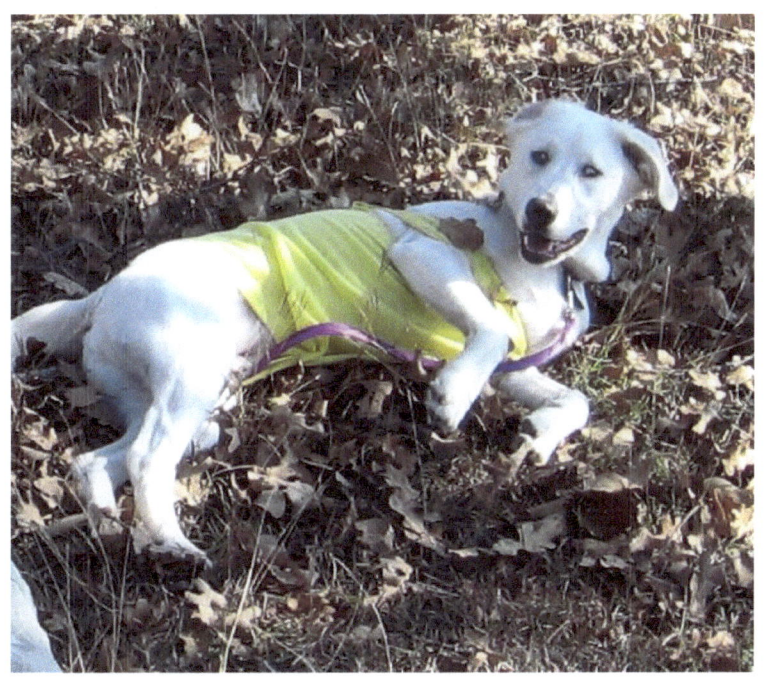

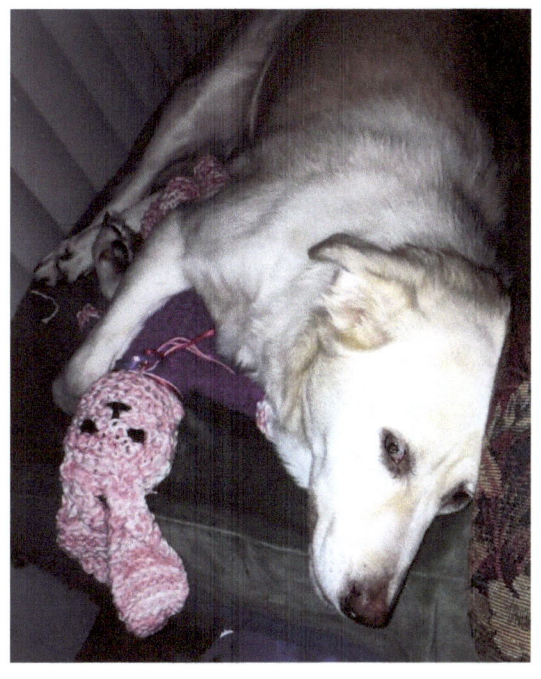

It's also very very important to remember to rest when you feel tired so that your body will be ready to play again tomorrow.

Mommy has to remind her friends
that they can't play rough
with her because it can
hurt her.
Sometimes she
must wear braces or
splints on her hands and
knees and ankles to
protect those joints
from getting dislocated.

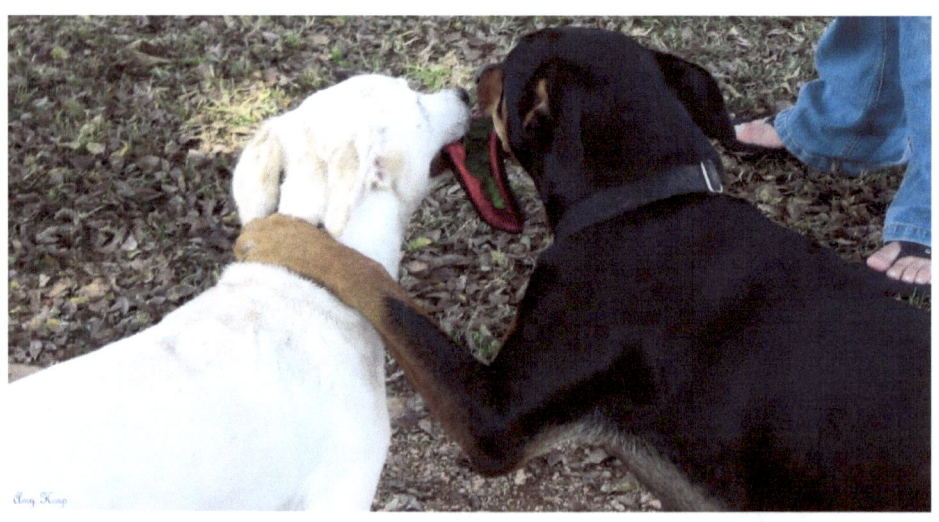

Having Ehlers Danlos Syndrome means that you have lots of health problems with your body.

It also means that you feel sick most of the time.

So sometimes you have to learn to do things a different way. My Mommy taught me how to do something special to help us on days when we don't feel well.

When I was a puppy, my Mommy taught me how to potty on special potty paper for dogs. She did this so she wouldn't have to take me outside to potty on the days that she feels sick and is in pain. I didn't do such a great job at first but then I finally caught on.

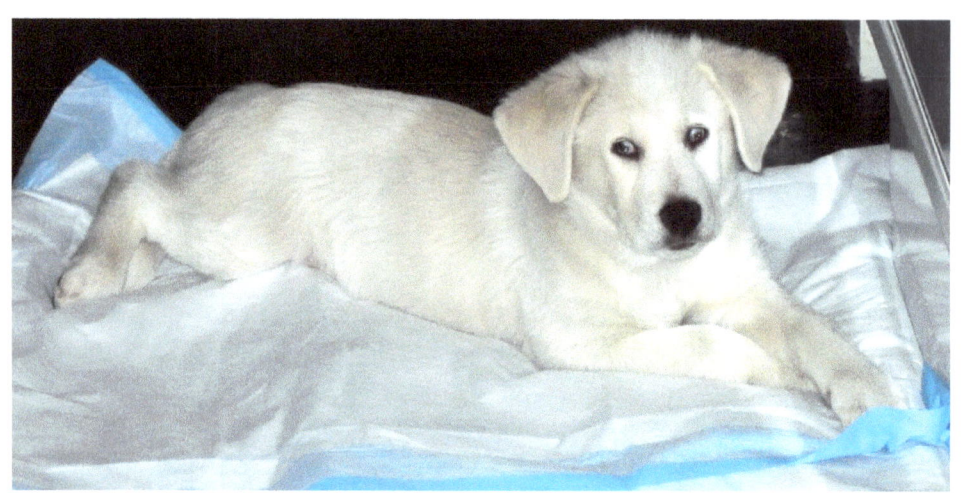

At first,
I just laid on
the potty paper.

Then I spent lots of time ripping it up
and spreading it all over the floor.

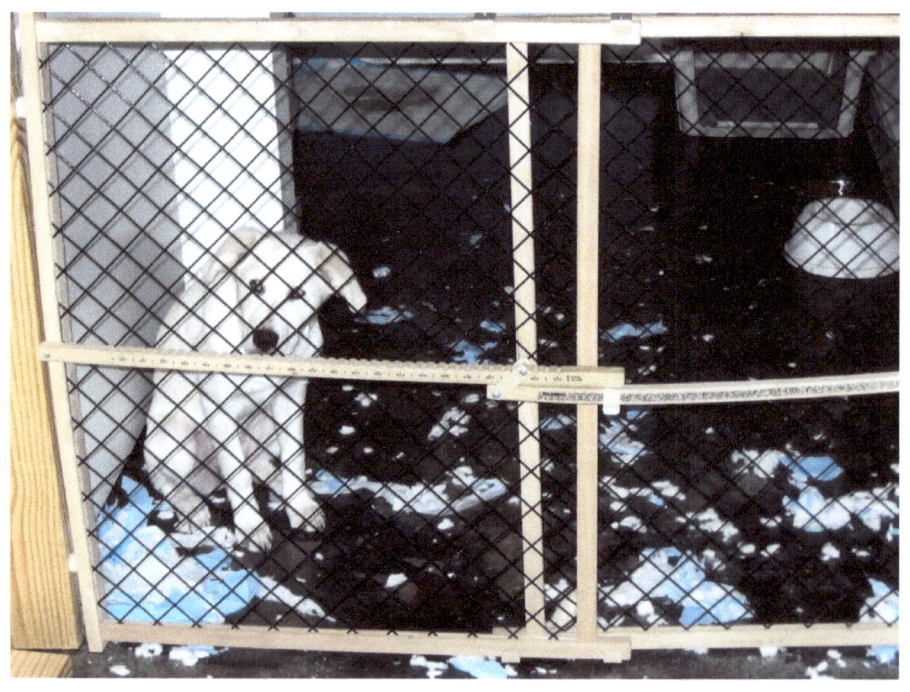

Mommy had to pick it up
and when she bent over to pick all
that paper up, she got dizzy.

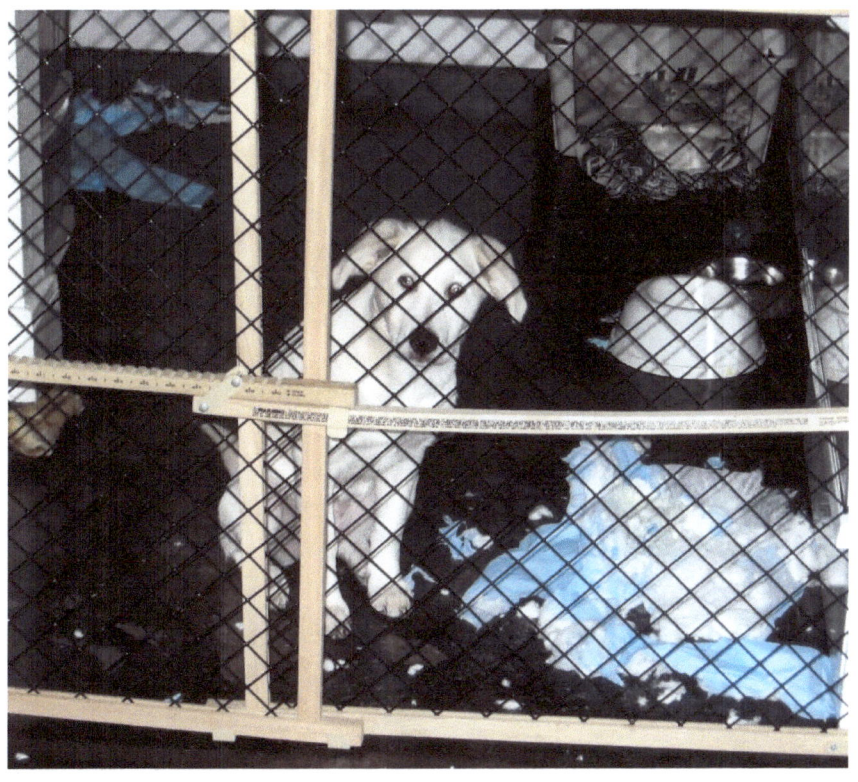

Getting dizzy happens a
lot when you have
EDS.

When I was a puppy and I ripped up my potty papers,
Mommy didn't get mad at me, she just told me to not do
that again and I didn't rip up my potty papers anymore.

I'm so good at using potty paper that no matter where we go Mommy brings some of the potty paper with us and she will put it on the floor and show me where it is and then when I need to potty, I know just what to do!

It has helped both of us for me to know how to use the potty paper because when it is extra cold or hot outside our bodies hurt and sometimes we have a hard time breathing because EDS can also make our lungs hurt.

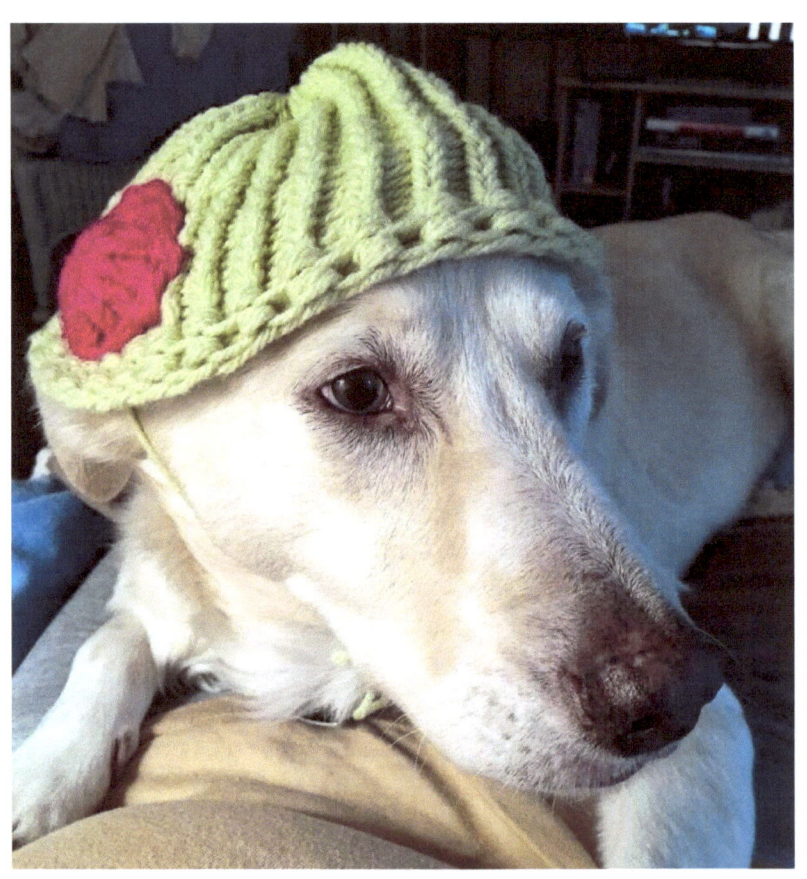

Mommy made a hat for me to wear when it's cold outside!

Mommy and I love spending time together
and there are many ways that
I help my Mommy.
Sometimes I help her
with her disabilities.

Some dogs learn how to help
people with disabilities. They are
trained to be a Service Dog.

After they are trained as a Service Dog they
can go anywhere their owner goes.
People will know which dogs are
Service Dogs because they
wear a special vest that lets
people know they are helping their owner.

There are lots of different disabilities that people can have besides EDS. Some people who have disabilities need extra help. That extra help sometimes comes
by way of a Service Dog.

Service Dogs are not allowed to be touched. Petting a service dog will take their attention away from their owner.
The owner is counting on their service dog
paying attention to the owner's needs.

A service dog is a dog who knows how to help their owner
do all kinds of things that are hard for them
to do on their own because of their owner's disability.

EDS is a disability that makes doing
normal everyday things hard.

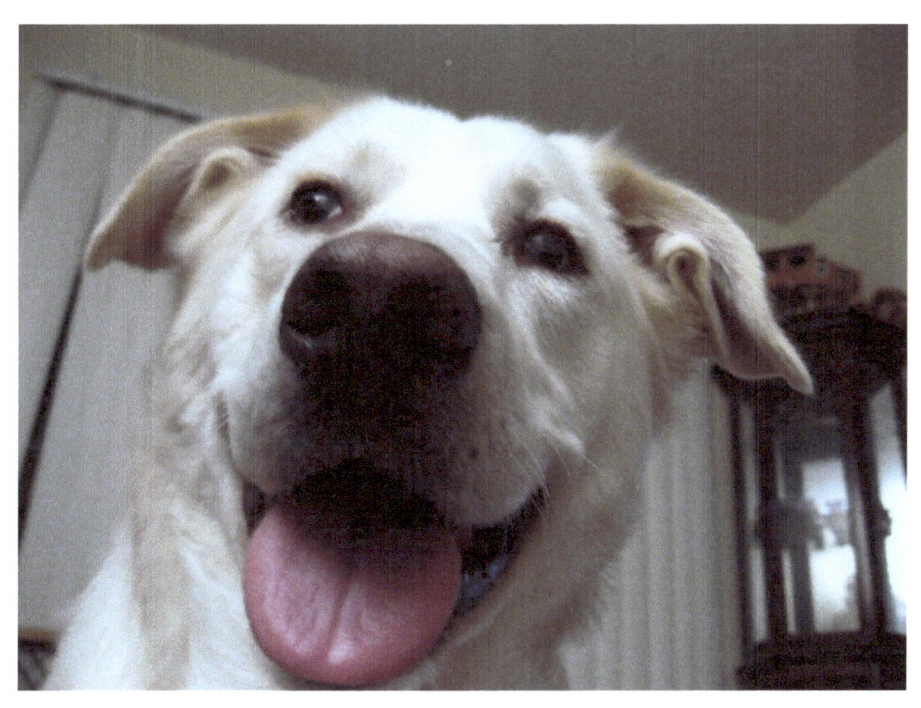

I get so happy when I get to go places with Mommy to help her.

I get to help Mommy because
I am a helping dog.

I am not a Service Dog; instead I am an Emotional Support Dog. I don't have to have the same training as a Service Dog. I'm not required to wear a special vest or any vest at all.

An Emotional Support Dog gives emotional support to their owner because they might be sad or scared when they need to have medical tests done at the hospital
or the doctor's office.

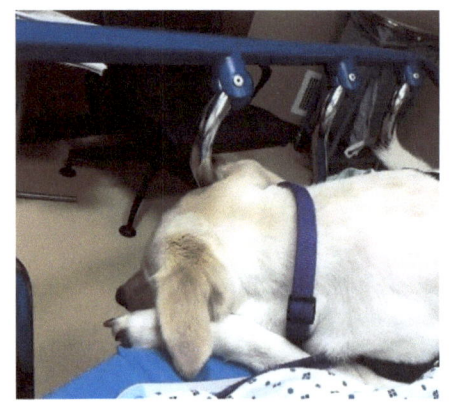

I give emotional support to my Mommy
by sitting close to her so she can
reach down and scratch my
head and ears, which I love!
Me being there helps
Mommy feel warm
inside and peaceful.

I also get to go grocery shopping with my Mommy. I sit on the cart for handicapped people right by Mommy's feet. I ride all around the store and I'm good at sitting still and watching the other people shopping.

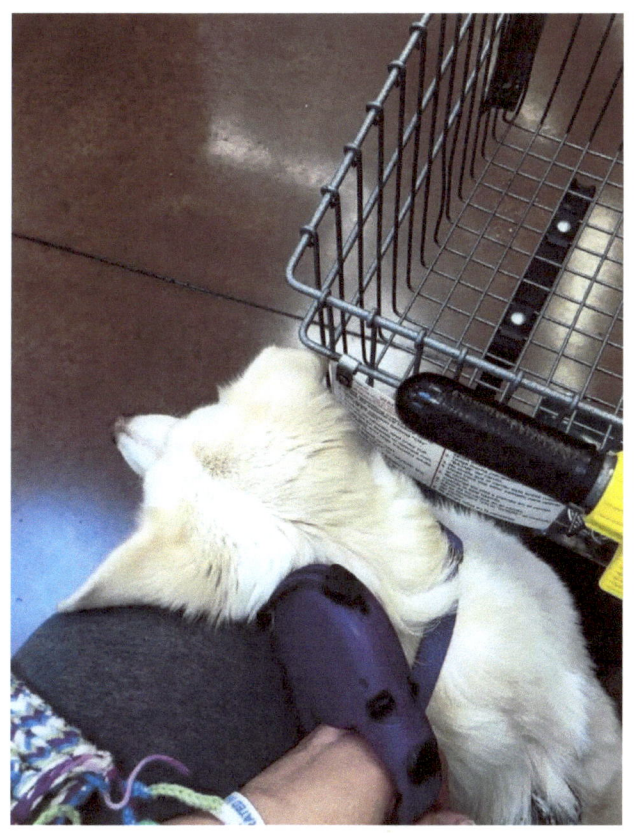

People always like to talk to me and pet me and that makes Mommy smile. It takes her mind off what is causing her pain and making her feel sick. People can pet me because I'm a support dog, not a service dog.

Ehlers Danlos Syndrome is hard to live
with at times and it does make my
Mommy and I have to live our lives
differently than most dogs and people who do not have EDS.

Mommy and I don't mind that very much
because we get to spend lots of time together.

One of the things that I can do
to help my Mommy is show her
in a special way just how much
I love her by going places with her
and helping her stay calm and feel loved.

Sometimes I do silly things
to help Mommy feel happy.
When I wear funny hats Mommy laughs.

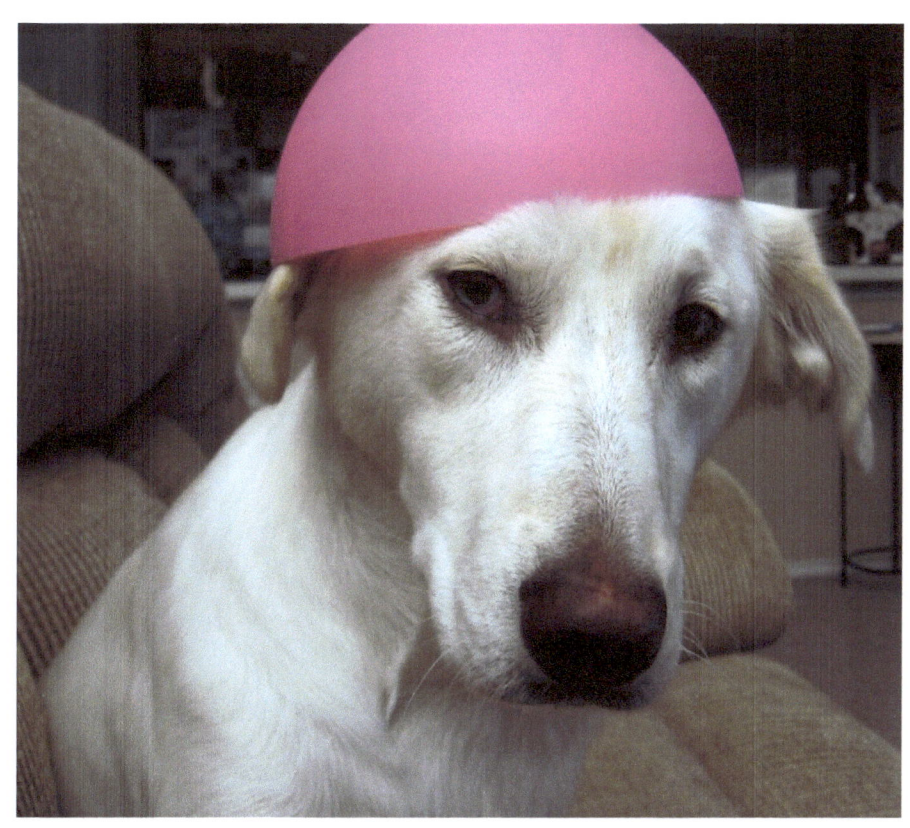

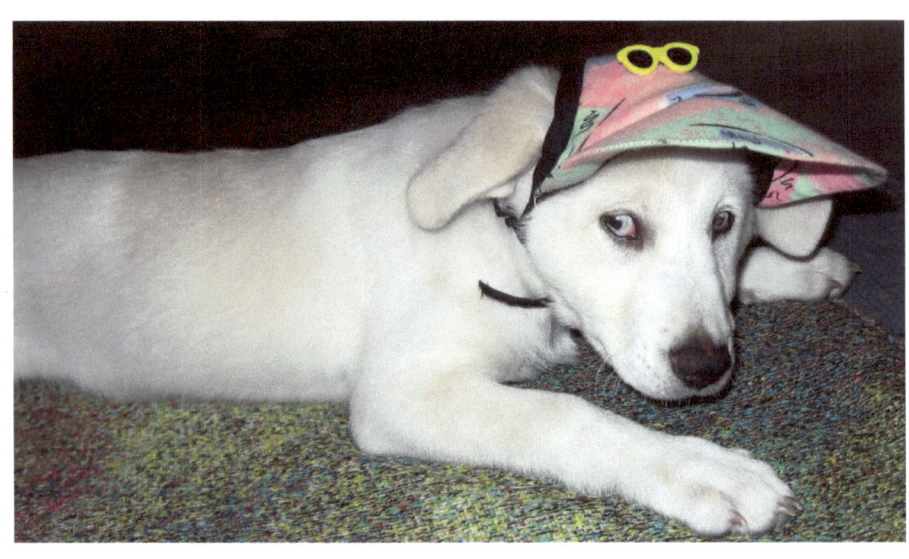

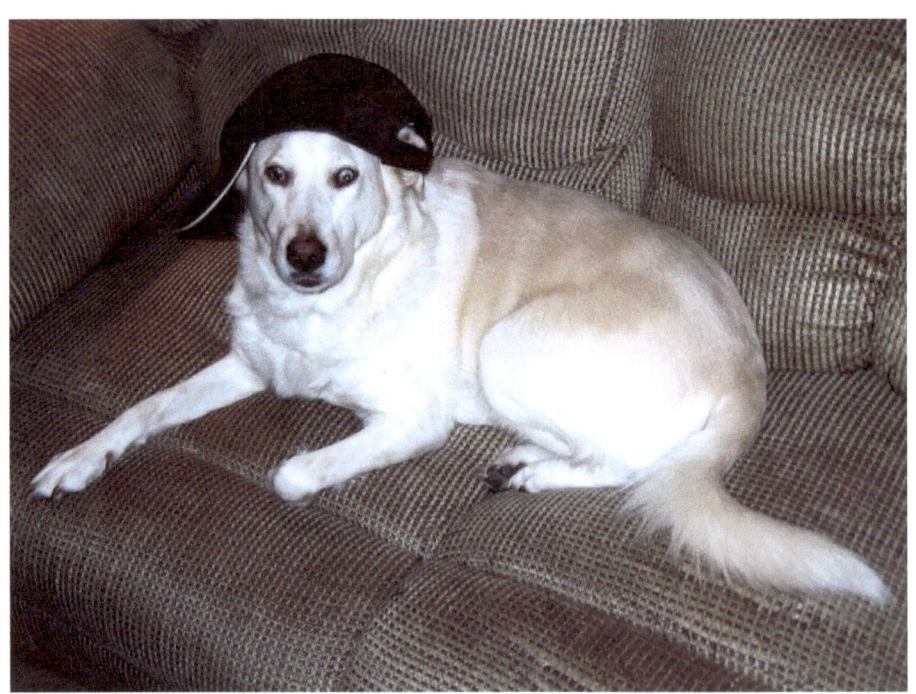

Sometimes I make silly faces to make Mommy laugh.

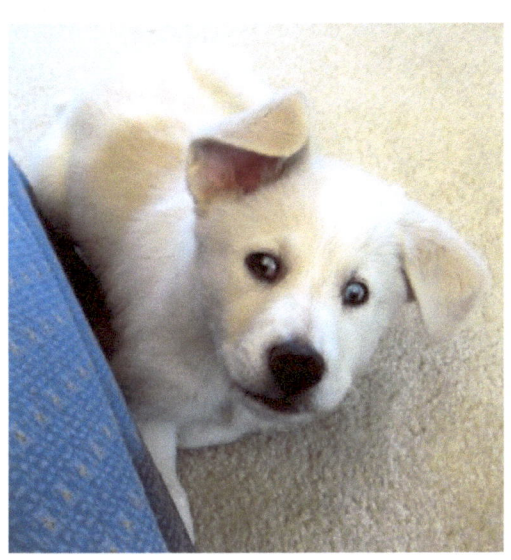

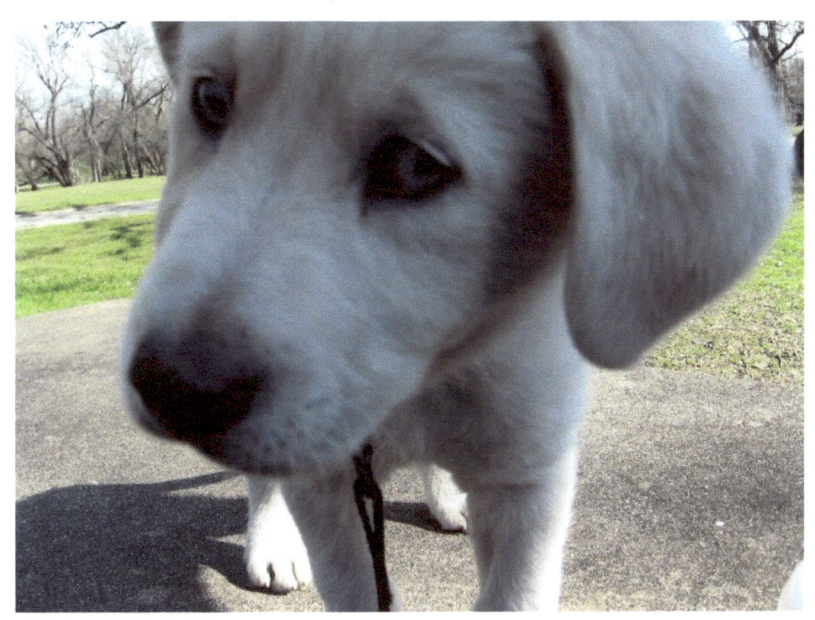

Other times I like to play keep away with my toys. Mommy laughs at how silly I get trying to keep my toys all to myself.

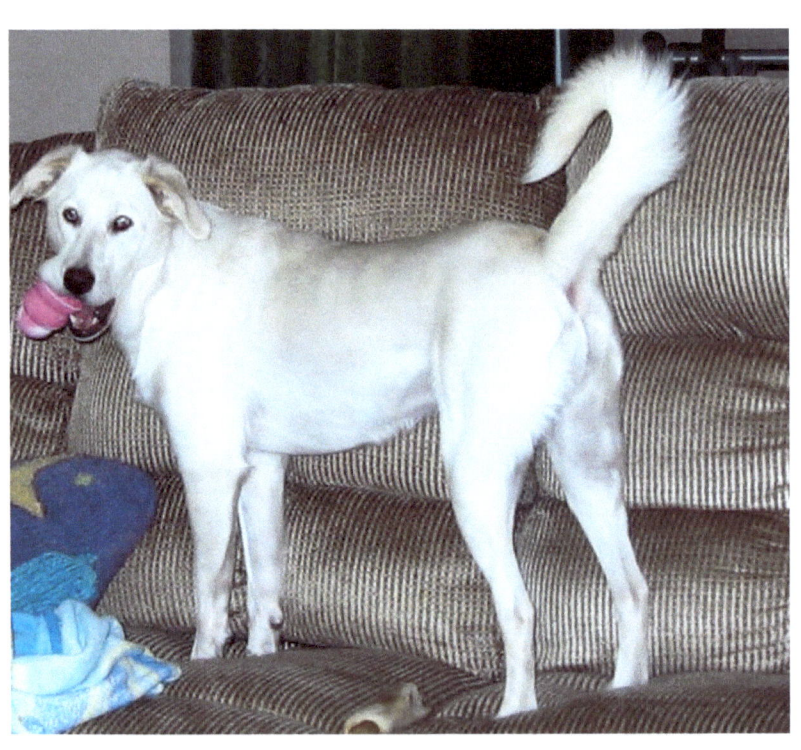

I love to watch out the window
to make sure I can report
to Mommy everything
going on outside.

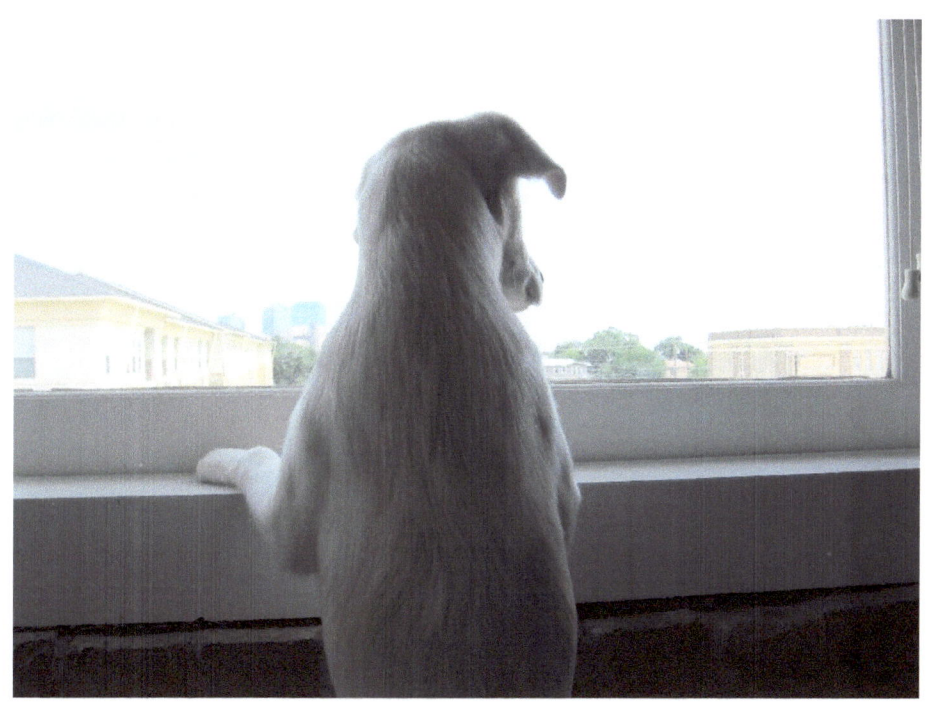

Most of all I am always ready to
help Mommy
whenever
she needs me.

I can't always put into barks
what I feel for my Mommy, but I sit
really close to her and sometimes curl
up in her lap and give her lots of
kisses and she gives me lots of kisses.

One more thing

that I can do for

Mommy is show her

with my paws that

I

Heart

my

Mommy!!!!

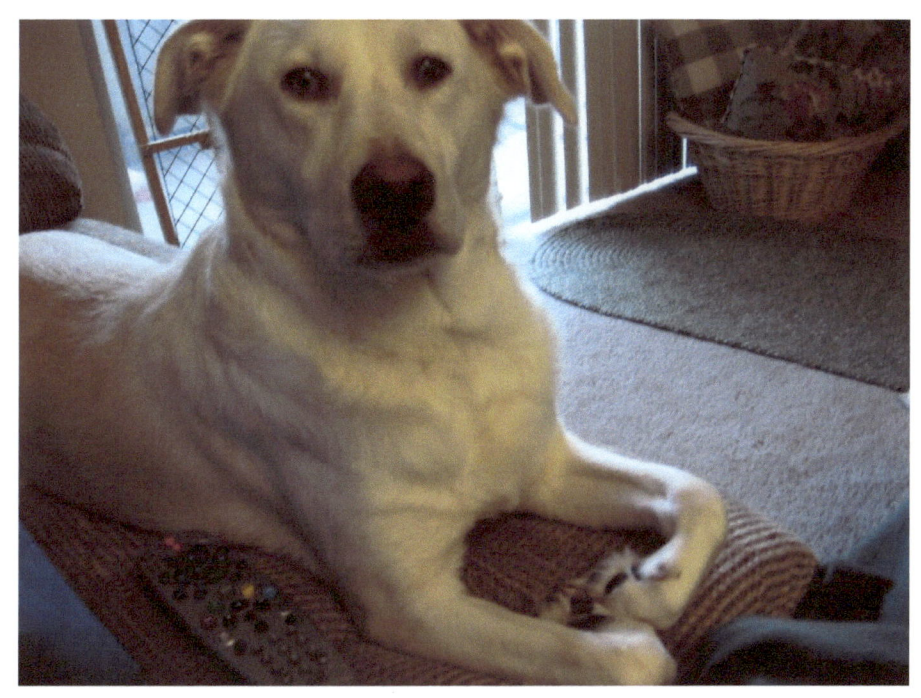

Look I made a heart with my paws!

To find out more about Ehlers Danlos Syndrome Please check out these websites:

www.genesthatdontfit.net

www.Prettyill.com

www.Medical@prettyill.com
(Medical and Healthcare Professionals only)

The Ehlers-Danlos Society - www.ehlers-danlos.com

EDS Awareness - www.chronicpainpartners.com

For any questions or inquiries for speaking engagements please call Amy Hosp at 214-476-1167

You can find Amy Hosp at:
www.genesthatdontfit.net
The Liberty Of It All:
www.thelibertyofitall.com

The Liberty of It All
With Genes That Don't Fit ©

You can purchase this book anywhere that books are sold online

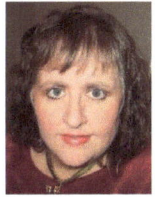

Bio

    Amy Hosp grew up in Frisco TX and she is a graduate of Dallas Christian College where she earned a B.S. in Ministry & Leadership, and has spent some time working toward earning a Master's degree at Southwestern Baptist Theological Seminary in Ft. Worth TX. In 2005 Amy served as a missionary in Nigeria.

    In 2012 Amy was diagnosed with a rare genetic disorder called Ehlers Danlos Syndrome Classical Type I and in 2018 another rare genetic disorder call Osteogenesis Imperfecta Type I. This extremely rare combination of genetic disorders causes a host of health issues that has left Amy disabled. Despite her disabilities Amy enjoys random adventures ranging from a spur of the moment road trip to the country, to exploring ideas of the unknown in life. Her life is a voyage and she wants to invite you to go along with her and find in you, what she has and is still finding, "The person that God created me to be!"

    Amy is a writer, photographer, musician and a missionary. She deals with life by always looking for the positive side to every situation and she will leave you with a smile. Her passion is to challenge the minds of others to look deep inside of themselves and look at life from a different perspective and also to find the true gifting's of God in their lives. Amy brings a unique view to understanding God's fullness and happiness for today's Christian believer.

Notes:

www.ingramcontent.com/pod-product-compliance
Lightning Source LLC
Chambersburg PA
CBHW051217220526
45473CB00003B/1068